WordTOOLS

For

Wellness

Vol. 2

Harnessing the
Power of Words!

Carol L Rickard, LCSW

Well YOUniversity® Publications

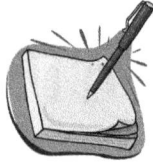

Sign up now!

To be sure to get our weekly motivational &
inspirational quotes and stories!

ThePowerOfWordsEQuote.com

ISBN-13: 978-1-947745-05-6

WordTools for Wellness Vol. 2

Harnessing the Power of Words!

by Carol L Rickard, LCSW

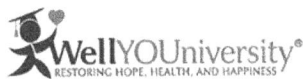

WellYOUniversity®
RESTORING HOPE, HEALTH, AND HAPPINESS

888 LIFE TOOLS (543-3866)

Carol@WellYOUniversity.com

Welcome!

My 1st WordTool came to me in 2006 when doing a group with my patients. How could I get them to *welcome* change in their lives?

Creating **H**ealthy **A**nd **N**ew **G**rowth **E**xperiences!

From there it's been an onward journey! Most of them are inspired by persons or situations. My hope is to create Ah-Ah moments that can help change a life!

They are officially called "Artinyms", which is Sanskrit for "describe".

On the back of each wordtool is a question for you. Answering them will serve to strengthen your wellness.

~To Living Well TODAY! ~

Carol

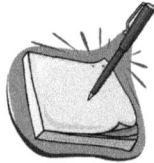

Sign up now!

To be sure to get our weekly motivational &
inspirational quotes and stories!

ThePowerOfWordsEQuote.com

A
Deliberate
Adjustment
Providing
Transformation

When is a time when you *adapted* and
how did it go?

Acquire

Self

Knowledge

What have you always wanted to know but were afraid to *ask*?

Adjusting

Thinking

To

Intentionally

Take

Us

Direction

Excellence

How would you describe your *attitude*?

Does it need adjusting?

Actively

Work

At

Recognizing

Existence

How would your life be different if you were more **aware** every day!

$\mathbf{C}$ounts

$\mathbf{A}$s

$\mathbf{N}$ot

‘

$\mathbf{T}$rying

What is it you have been telling yourself that you *CAN'T* do? Have you even tried?

Creating

Healthy

And

New

Growth

Experiences

What are some important *changes* you could make in your life that would pay off BIG?

$$\textbf{C}\text{reate}$$

$$\textbf{A}$$

$$\textbf{L}\text{evel}$$

$$\textbf{M}\text{indset}$$

What are some of the areas in your life where you need more *clarity*?

Cultivating

A

Responsive

Environment

When was a time you made a **compromise**?

What was the outcome?

Concentrate

On

Not

Stopping

Instead

Strengthening

The

Effort

Needed

Today

What do you need to be *consistent* with that has been difficult for you to do in the past?

Direct

Opportunity

Do you have any *debt* in your life?

How is it impacting your life?

Denied

Opportunity

Not

'

Trying!

What is it that you still want to **DO** in your
lifetime?

Dwelling

On

Unfounded

Beliefs &

Thoughts

What has *doubt* stopped you from doing?

What would you do if it didn't exist?

Engage

Full

Force

On

Reaching

Targets

What are some goals you have that could use some *effort* towards?

Extremely

Valuable

Activity

Letting

Us

Assess

True

Effectiveness

Do you tend to be someone who *evaluates* decisions? What have you learned?

Fully

Examine

Emotional

Lessons

Are there any *facts* you are facing a hard time trying to deal with?

Find

An

Important

Lesson

Using

Real

Experiences

What are some important lessons you have
learned from *failure*?

Fix

Our

Concentration

Until

Successful

What are you planning to use your *focus* to achieve?

Giving

Respect

And

Thanks

Everyday

For

Unbelievable

Life!

Make a list of all the things you are *grateful* for having in your life:

$\mathbf{G}$radually

$\mathbf{R}$ecognize

$\mathbf{O}$ur

$\mathbf{W}$ay

What are some of the ways in which you have *grown* over the last year? Last 5 years?

Incredible

Mental

Activity

Generating

Ideas

Not

Existing!

If you were to let It run wild, what would you *imagine* your life to look like 1 year from now?

I

Now

See

Possibility

In

Reaching &

Engaging

Daily

Who have been some of the people in your life
that have *inspired* you?

Link

Education

And

Resources

Needed!

What is it that you don't know how to do that you'd like to *learn*?

Moments

Intentionally

Noticed

Directly

Fixing

Unconscious

Living

What steps are you taking to *market*? Who is your established target customer?

Necessary

Elements

Enabling

Daily

Survival

What are your life *needs*?

What are your business's needs?

Purposely

Laid

Activity

Necessary

Succeed

Do you have any *plans* for the coming year?
If so, what are they? If not, why not?

Personal

Experience

Empowered

Recovery

What is the opportunity you have to share with others? What's stopping you from *promoting*?

Release

Emotions

And

Create

Trouble

When was a time in your life where you *reacted* & made the situation worse?

Result

Is

Seldom

Known

What are you willing to *risk* in the pursuit of success?

Swiftly

Take

Action

Reaching

Targets

What have been some of the actions or goals you
have not *started* yet?

To

Risk

Uncertainty

Seeking

Togetherness

What does a person need to show you in order for you to **trust** them?

About the Author

Carol L Rickard, LCSW, TTS, of Hopewell, NJ is founder & CEO of WellYOUniversity, LLC, a global health education company dedicated *to empowering individuals with the tools and supports to achieve lifelong wellness & recovery.*

Also known as *America's Wellness Ambassador*, Carol is a dynamic & engaging speaker who brings to life practical / useful solutions. She is a weekly contributor for Esperanza Magazine; written 13 books on stress and wellness, had a guest appearance on Dr. Oz last year

She is also the creator & host of a 30-minute wellness show on Princeton TV - **The WELL YOU Show** which current episodes are aired on Mondays at 6:00pm EST & Sundays at 8:30am EST and can be watched at PrincetonTV.org.

All episodes available at: **www.TheWELLYOUShow.com**

Get more of Carol at:

Twitter: ***@wellYOUlife***

"Like us" @ www.FaceBook.com/WellYOUniversity

Have Carol Speak at Your Next Event!

Get more information about how you can have Carol speak at your organization, event, or conference.

Go to: www.CarolLRickard.com

Or call: 888 Life Tools (543-3866)

Carol's Other Books

Getting Your Mind to Mind You

ANGER – A Simple & Practical Approach

Help – How to Help Those Who DON'T Want it

Selfness – Simple Self-Care Secrets

Stress Eating – How to STOP Using Food to Cope

Stretched Not Broken – Caregiver's Stress

The Caregiver's Toolbox

Transforming Illness to Wellness

Putting Your Weight Loss on Auto

The Benefits of Smoking

Moving Beyond Depression

LifeTools – How to Manage Life

Creating Compliance

Relapse Prevention

Please visit us at:

www.WellYOUniversity.com

Sign up for weekly motivational e-quote!

Check out our upcoming FREE webinars!

Learn more about our training programs.

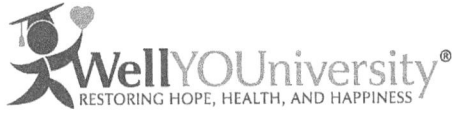

Email us your success story at:

Success@WellYOUniversity.com

We'd like to ask for your feedback

Please check out the next page
if this book has been HELPFUL for you!

We'd love to hear from you!

Feedback Card

Please take a moment & provide us some
feedback about the book you just read &
how you feel *it benefited YOU!*

_____

_____

_____

_____

Name: _____

Best Phone #: _____

Can we use your comments in our publicity materials?
Yes / No

If OK with you, what's the best time to call you:_____

Thank You!

Scan or take a picture & email:
Carol@WellYOUniversity.com

Snail mail: Carol Rickard
5 Zion Rd., Hopewell, NJ 08535

Tear along here